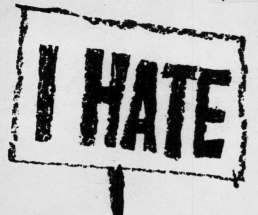

the **to exercise book**

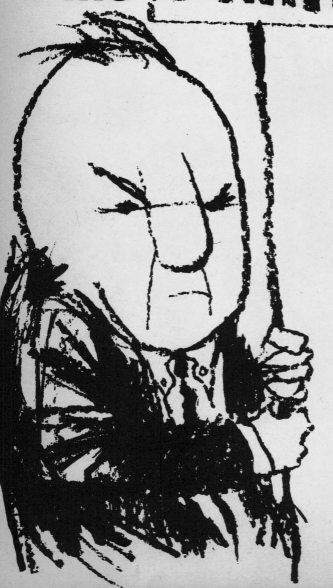

to exercise book

BY STEPHEN HUFFAKER

ILLUSTRATIONS BY CHARLES FELLOWS

CORNERSTONE LIBRARY · NEW YORK

CORNERSTONE LIBRARY PUBLICATIONS
are distributed by
Simon & Schuster, Inc.
630 Fifth Avenue, New York, N.Y. 10020
Lithographed in the United States of America
under the supervision of
Rolls Offset Printing Co., Inc., N.Y.

CONTENTS

PREFACE

This program takes only five minutes a day, certainly not very long to accomplish the difficult job of keeping oneself fit; but let me assure you, it's enough.

The magic involved in this method, if there is any, lies in its simplicity. Maybe a better word would be practicality. I have found that most exercise programs are too difficult. They require too much discipline to stay with them. My aim is to eliminate a major part of that discipline so that you will reap the benefits of exercise because it will be easy for you to do.

I have no quarrel with other exercise programs. Indeed, I have never known a single one that I did not find extremely beneficial. Exercise *IS* beneficial, and I am for it in every way. My challenge is merely that most exercise programs are made too difficult for the average individual whose most strenuous regular pursuit will be a short run to the train after an average day's work.

In other words:

MOST PHYSICAL FITNESS PROGRAMS HAVE NOT BEEN AIMED AT THE PEOPLE WHO NEED THEM MOST!

My theory is simply this: a little exercise done over a long period is more beneficial to your body than a lot of exercise done over a short period, interrupted by long periods of complete inactivity. The basis of this theory lies in the fact that the body functions better when it functions with regularity. Consider other ways in which this theory is borne out:

7

(1) Normally gradual dieting is better for the body than a "crash" diet.

(2) Our digestive process would function better, and more food energy would be transformed directly to usable body energy, if we would eat less food more often. Say, five or six small meals rather than three large ones.

(3) It is more refreshing to our bodies to sleep shorter periods, more often. Because the best sleep comes immediately after we fall asleep, it would be more beneficial to sleep, say, five hours at night, get up earlier, and take a nap in the afternoon.

The control of some of these "more natural" body functions is not possible because of our work and social commitments. But it *is* possible to control an exercise program, and that is what I have attempted to do. I have tried to draw a compromise between human will-power and human fitness.

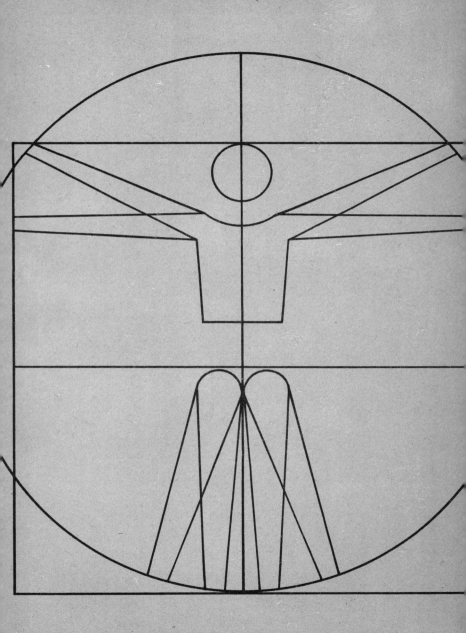

9

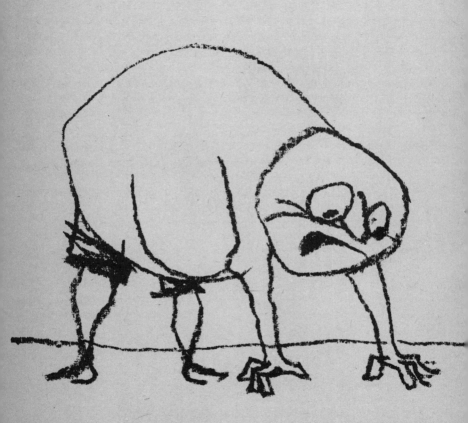

Chapter **1**

EXERCISE IS A DIRTY WORD

While serving as a physical training instructor in the Air Force one fact of my work stood out above all others— FEW PEOPLE LIKE TO EXERCISE! We are unanimous in our desire for the benefit; it's just the exercise itself that we don't like.

Is it some comfort to know that we are not alone in our lack of regard for exercise? In fifteen years of association with athletic teams and physical fitness programs of all kinds, I have yet to find one person who really likes doing individual exercises, just for the enjoyment that exercise brings.

The reason is simple. Exercise requires EXERTION, and in any language that means work.

WHAT IS EXERCISE?

As a new physical training instructor my idea of conditioning exercises was that of a well-disciplined group of people, smartly executing the drills under a hot sun, complete with snappy cadence count and youthful high-spirited morale. But over the years I began to realize that this wasn't realistic exercise at all, but rather a crash program of torture that no human could possibly continue. And what was more unrealistic, this type of strenuous activity was only meant for the young, the active,

11

the healthy—not at all suitable for those of us who really need it.

Not that I mean to call the majority of us old, lazy, and ailing. It's just that it doesn't make sense to think we are something that we aren't.

So let's face facts. Most of us are human. We eat too much. We drink too much. We smoke too much. And *exercise* is a dirty word; it's too hard and takes too much discipline.

WATCH OUT FOR RATIONALIZATION

"If a little extra fat is the price I have to pay for enjoying the luxuries of life, then I'll just have to pay it."

No, it's not that simple either. We really don't enjoy being overweight, short of breath, and susceptible to every little painful strain and pull that catches the unused muscle and joint. We don't really enjoy the extra effort it takes to do the little things; roll over in bed, tie our shoe, pick up the newspaper. Even exiting from the car is somewhat like being born again. No, and we don't enjoy knowing that all of it will catch up with us one day, and slice an undecided amount of time off our lives. But if we're being honest, let's consider both sides.

So exercise is somewhat like the seatbelts in our car. Of course they're good, but the discomfort of their use when totaled through the years may be greater than the hardship they are designed to prevent. That's a good point. Let me draw an analogy from it. If we could get into our car, buckle our seatbelt and then by some miraculous happening become totally unaware of its existence, wouldn't it make a difference? It wouldn't restrict our movement, cramp our legs, or make us feel out of place when nobody else used theirs. We would feel more inclined to use them because they had become easier to use!

That's the same thought I had about exercise. People neglect doing them because for most people they are more trouble than they are worth. And just like with seatbelts, the only known alternative is to give them up altogether. So I looked for an easier way, a way to derive a good share of the benefits, without suffering the torture of the task. Thus, this practical exercise program.

NOT A CURE-ALL

It's a very simple program, but before I tell you what it is, I'll admit to you what it is not. It's not a cure-all for everything that ails you, anymore than an aspirin will cure a cold. If you engage in physical over-exertion, like the annual game of softball at the company picnic, your muscles will still tell you about it the next day. It will not keep you slim, nor does it promise any "miraculous" transfiguration of natural body shape. In short, YOU supply the benefits that you derive from this program just as you would any other method of exercise. The big difference is that these exercises are easy, practical, and tailored for you—so that you get the benefit YOU need and not what someone else wants you to have.

Now, here's what this simple program will do. It will all but eliminate shortness of breath. It will exercise and condition the commonly used muscles so that you will be free from the strains and pulls that plague the inactive. Your midsection will stay within the limit to permit mobility for stretching and stooping. Your back and spine will have the "athlete's feel" of good health, allowing better rest and harder work. And your body will be far more resistant to illness, disease, and abuse, because of its increased state of strength and health.

THE HOOKER?

And what do you give in return for these benefits? Well, this program takes less than five minutes each day, and is done in the privacy of your own bathroom. It is quicker than a shave or a facial, and it treats your whole body. Even more, it treats your whole day. And it's as enjoyable as this task can be—most people say "ultra easy."

NOT FOR THE ATHLETE

Let me repeat that this book is not written for the athlete or the person who is already active. It is for the average human being, the one hundred million or so Americans who have no fitness program at all. Like any fitness program it is not for those who have medical problems that restrict physical exercise. Your doctor should give you the okay before undertaking any fitness program when a medical problem is involved.

I recently administered this program to an athlete, with the following results: Before the exercises, at rest, his pulse rate measured 74 per minute. *AFTER* the group of exercises it had increased to only 96. For all practical purposes it did him no good at all because it never reached his already achieved point of fitness. He was accustomed to doing "more" than these exercises in his daily work or play routine.

But for the great majority of us it is different. This book is written for the AVERAGE human being, and takes into consideration our average human frailties. It reverses the trend that has long been the downfall of most exercise programs, by making it as EASY as possible. Its aim is not to make you fit as an athlete, but rather, JUST FIT TO LIVE.

Chapter 2

WHY SHOULD WE EXERCISE?

THE FUEL WE BURN

Have you ever taken notice of the tremendous care that most owners give to their new automobile? I saw a beautiful example just the other day at the garage. A fat man of about forty was not content to wait in the customer's room while his car was being serviced. He peered intently under the hood as the serviceman worked to make sure that everything was done in the proper manner. He watched to insure that every part was lubricated sufficiently, and examined the cans of new oil carefully before allowing them to be put into the car. He smiled with pleasure when he was assured by the man that it was the best that money could buy. I took a moment to chat with him, telling him how nice his car looked and how obvious it was that he took good care of it. He swelled with pride as he recounted its performance and assured me that it paid great dividends to keep it in top shape to prevent anything from causing trouble later on.

I smiled as I thought how typical it was. "What a pity," I said to myself, "that he doesn't give his own body machine half the consideration that he gives to his car." The same man takes little note of the quality of the goods that go into his own crankcase.

OUR BODY MACHINE

The human body is a much finer machine than even the most expensive automobile. It will continually take any abuse we give it and do its best to function for us at our command. It repairs minor aches and pains on its own and never gives one word of complaint until the damage becomes so urgent that it needs our help to mend it. But

15

because it is so uncomplaining, we merely tend to abuse it more.

What if we had a playback of all the things that went into our body in the course of just one week? Cookies, candy, whiskey, gravies, spices, fats, hot coffee, cold soda, cakes, pies, ice cream, puddings, french fries, wine, spaghetti sauce, cigarette smoke, dressings, canapes, Chinese food, and......well, the list could go on and on. And note that these are only the things we would likely be better off without.

If we read a book on health it would probably say, "limit the amount of butter you consume each day; spread butter only thick enough to taste it and no more." Are you likely to take that advice? Of course not, unless you are aiming at a super-excellent body-building program. Another may say, "avoid all pastries, ice cream, pies, jams, jellies, all fried, fatty, and greasy foods, candy, sundaes, syrups, cereals, creamed soups and sauces, relishes, pickles, spiced meats, and white flour." Are you likely to take that advice? We both, you and I, know it's good advice, but will you take it? Of course not—it's too drastic, too hard.

Tomorrow evening on the way home from work you will stop at your favorite bar and have a beer. It takes the edge off the day and the few minutes of companionship with old friends eases your anxieties a bit before you report home to the family. You plan on only having one or two but the boys buy you another and slap you on the back. Are you going to turn it down? Of course not. It wouldn't be right if you did.

When you arrive at home your wife has a martini all made for you and tells you to sit down and rest before dinner. After a large, tender steak she surprises you with your favorite dessert, strawberry shortcake. Will you turn it down? Of course not, how could you?

WE ARE VICTIMS OF OUR AGE

Now the point is coming all too clear. We are certainly victims of the age and environment in which we live. Many of the delicacies that we enjoy today were not even heard of even 25 years ago. The variety of rich food and drink we have at our table is seemingly limited only by the limits of man's imagination. Likewise the variety of conveniences at our fingertips; autos, buses, dishwashers, automatic equipment of every description. What has happened to the lost art of manual labor? We get it both ways then, don't we? Not only do we have the richest eating habits of any country in the world, but our advances in technology have doubled the complexity of our problem.

ATTACKING THE PROBLEM

I told you earlier that we would look for the EASIEST way to attack the problem. So, why choose exercise?

We must choose exercise for several basic reasons. First, it is the only means of fitness that is solely in OUR hands. As we just pointed out, the social pressures we must face at times limit the control we have over the intake of our food and drink, and the temptation to abandon our will-power is much greater. Second, although by proper diet we could successfully control our weight problem, we would still be lacking in fitness and strength. Hence, we would still be in need of an exercise program. Let me reiterate once again that we would be better off if we could combine the two, diet and exercise, but we have already decided that you have only a limited amount of tolerance for this type of thing. So "maximum effect from minimum effort" is our watchword, and "exercise" is our means to that end.

PHYSICAL FITNESS AND EMOTIONAL STABILITY

I'm glad you see it that way because only with exercise, the dynamic movement of the muscles of the body, can you achieve the maximum benefit of not only the time you spend with this program, but of all your time, both waking and sleeping. The fitness we achieve through the physical condition of our bodies is not wholly mani-

17

fested in a "physical" way. In fact, a large part of "physical" fitness has its outlet in the "emotional" spectrum of our performance. When we are physically fit we feel less strain, less fatigue; we are able to cope more easily with extra burdens and stresses. When we feel better physically we have a completely different outlook on life, an improved attitude which will manifest itself in our every action, emotional or physical. You know this is true from personal experience. You can't work or act your best when something is bothering you physically. After the malady leaves, you feel better toward yourself and everything you do. Further, as your body increases its physical fitness, your mental and emotional health increases with it.

TRY THESE SIMPLE EXERCISES

Let me give you a couple of simple examples of how physical exercise helps your emotional condition. Lift your eyes from the book and do this exercise with them. While holding your head straight forward, run your eyes as far to the left and right as possible, even farther than you can see. Make them dart quickly back and forth, using the corners of your vision that you seldom use. Now run them up to the ceiling and to the floor and around in circles—give your eyes a good lively workout for just about 15 seconds. Now when you have done that, what have you noticed about your face. Don't your eyes almost force a smile upon your face? That's because you made them feel healthy, gave them something new and different to do. They liked the feeling and are sending that notice to your brain. Try that same exercise again sometime when your eyes are tired from overuse and see how it eases the strain.

Here's another. Take one hand and grasp the wrist of the other arm tightly. Now rotate the free hand around in all directions as far as it will go, both ways, backward and forward, to the sides. It will crack and snap a little, but that won't hurt it. When you're through (just ten seconds or so) lay your hand on your lap or a table and note the good feeling of life in it. Think about your hand and see how good it feels. Now lift your foot off the floor and do the same thing with your foot and ankle. Just on its own, run the foot around in circles, both ways, as far as it will reach. Feels good, doesn't it? Try it tomorrow when you awake and see how refreshing it is.

EXERCISE STIMULATES YOUR BODY

Yes, exercise stimulates the life in your body. The tissues wake up and ask to serve you because you have awakened them, and have given them something to do. Remember the good feeling your tired feet used to get when you stood on the vibrator machine in the corner drugstore or at the amusement park. Or how you have languished under the smooth, strong hands of a masseur as he worked the stiffness out of those unused joints and muscles. That too, is a form of exercise, and although it feels good, what you do in your own home is better and more beneficial.

YOUR WORK CAPACITY INCREASES

Physical fitness through exercise is merely the increasing of your capacity to perform work by letting the not-so-often-used muscles of your body increase their activity and effectiveness. As the inactive muscles and organs learn to perform more work, they become more efficient and you become healthier. Even outstanding athletes are faced with the problem of reconditioning muscles. I have observed it hundreds of times on athletic fields and gymnasiums throughout the country. Put an athlete, no matter how good he is, on the field after a long layoff and observe him closely. You will soon see that his mind reacts faster than his body because his muscles have lapsed into a lesser degree of activity. You will see his surprise as his eyes reach for the ball but his arms and legs don't follow. He misses a play that used to be easy for him to make. He must recondition his muscles through use, to achieve the efficiency they once knew.

In our own, lesser way, we are no different. Our muscles become tight and stiff through non-use, and one day it dawns on us that we can't bend like we once could, can't reach like we once could. We're rusty, stiff, and we need a little loosening. After a few weeks of exercise we can feel the simple chores begin to come easier. Our legs and back become more supple and bend to the task with ease. Not only that, but our internal organs, heart and lungs are stronger and are functioning a good deal easier under their newly acquired capacity. Of course the results of this new health and strength are obvious. Our resistance to many kinds of illness is much higher, and our capacity to sustain an illness and bounce back to good health is faster and greater.

EXERCISE "SAVES" US TIME

Now, remember that we have been talking about efficiency. We know, of course, that efficiency means time. The more easily we do a job, the longer we can stay at it, or the less energy we spend doing the same task. Either way, we have either saved time, or put out more work in a given length of time. That's an important point to us because our time is valuable, at least to us. I make this point because I want to show you that the five minutes of time you give to yourself in the morning building your strength will not only be beneficial to you in increased physical and emotional fitness, but will return many times its value in actual time saved through efficiency of movement and thus greater personal effectiveness.

I have taken the time to explain the logic behind our exercise program because I want to be sure that you understand what we are doing, and why we are doing it. If I have settled that question in your mind we will move on to the next point which deals with where we will actually perform our exercises.

Chapter 3

WHERE TO EXERCISE

RAREFOOT IN THE PARK

I watched as the runner came around the corner of the park to my right and strode evenly along the huge expanse of grass directly in front of me. He was dressed in running gear; gray shorts, red and white T-shirt, and low-cut running shoes. It was obvious by his confidence that he had been there many times, but one could still detect an intentional improvement in his style as he passed in view of the scores of people lining the path and benches where I sat. All eyes were on him for the few minutes it took to negotiate along the right-hand perimeter and disappear through the trees at the far end, where he could run in comparative privacy for a couple of hundred yards before he would reappear once again on our left.

He likely was a trackman, running in the park to escape the boredom of countless laps around an oval track. But maybe not. Maybe he was taking a workout in the park to get himself into better shape, or just to feel better! He looked in good condition so I rather think that he was the former. If he hadn't looked in good condition, and he hadn't looked good running, I wonder if he would have been out there in public? I didn't think so then, and I don't think so now.

RUNNING IS TOPS

Running is one of the best exercises we can do, probably the BEST single exercise. It's natural, working the muscles and organs the way they were intended to be worked. And it gets to the heart of physical fitness, deep into the lungs, and other internal organs that so seldom get their share of conditioning. But I don't even have to ask the question. I know without asking that I'm not going to get YOU out and running in the park! It's difficult enough when you're young, trim, and run well, but *now* the thought is absurd. It's pretty difficult to look incognito when you're 40 pounds overweight and sniffing and lumbering around the park. The vultures would likely fly circular patterns over your path, waiting for you to drop dead.

RUNNING-IN-PLACE

But running and jogging is still one of the best exercises we can do—so we'll do a little of it. Not in the park, but in the privacy of our own home. Before you start moving the furniture around in preparation for a track, let me console you further. You won't move a foot, we'll do our running IN PLACE.

Running-in-place may not seem as glamorous as the conventional style, and you won't find many young athletes who care for it at all. But the fact remains that running-in-place uses exactly the same muscles and organs as free running and gives us exactly the same benefit. Don't get me wrong, running-in-place slowly doesn't give us the same conditioning as running fast. But running-in-place slowly does give us the same conditioning as running slowly or jogging, and running-in-place at a faster pace gives us the same conditioning as running fast.

IN THE BATHROOM

Of course you may do the exercises in this book anywhere you desire, but I would like you to consider doing them in your bathroom. The reason I say this is because I will talk to you later about developing the HABIT of doing these simple exercises daily, and so I think we should pick a place where it's easiest to start and develop a habit. I don't know your daily schedule or what you may be doing at any given time of the day. But I do know that most of you get up in the morning, and that seems a good starting point. In addition, you are well-rested and will do them easier, and in turn, they will help waken you and liven the start of your day.

Now, why the bathroom instead of your bedroom? Simply, the bathroom is usually the most private place in your house. I realize that many of you will laugh about this when you have four kids, a wife, and a dog waiting in line for the bathroom at 7:20 in the morning, but don't give up the idea without a try, and I'll tell you why.

FITNESS IS PERSONAL BUSINESS

YOUR physical condition is YOUR personal business. If you're fifty pounds overweight it may be embarrassing to do exercises in front of other people, even your own family. You may privately want to achieve better conditioning without letting anyone know about it. You may not want to let others know what bad shape you have let yourself get into. These reasons sound simple, but I know that they have been stumbling blocks to others before, and so I offer them to you.

I knew a fellow who felt bad about the condition of his body and decided to do something about it. He carried on a vigorous program of exercises in the privacy of his bathroom every morning without one member of his family ever knowing it. He merely let it be known that he enjoyed long showers, completing his exercises while the noise of the shower drowned out any noise of the exercises. He wasted a little water, but he wasted away a lot of fat, too.

Regardless of the crowded condition of your household I contend that each of you can allot yourselves 12 minutes of privacy each morning in the bathroom. That is sufficient time to do your exercises, shave, and shower—and it's probably no more time than you're now taking.

Give it a try.

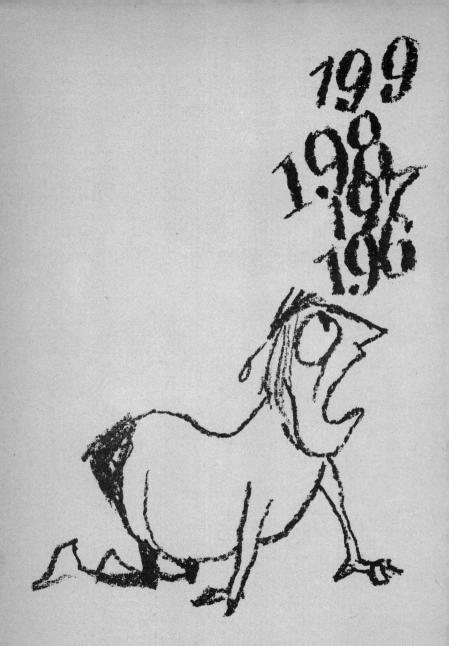

Chapter 4

HOW MUCH SHOULD WE EXERCISE?

Our existence is frequently a choice of extremes. We work too hard, we rest too much; we don't have enough money and we suffer from a lack of necessities, or we have too much and we suffer from rich living; our skin is pale from want of sunshine, or we over-expose ourselves and sustain a burn. The list is endless. Life is a constant battle of the opposites. It is difficult to achieve moderation because there are so many forces pulling at us from every side.

It's the same with exercise. The next most common fault after our resistance to doing any exercise at all is our tendency to overdo once we have begun. Overexertion, especially for the previously inactive or those just starting a program of exercise, can be just as harmful as the final effects of no exercise at all.

TAKE IT EASY

Don't be in a hurry to do something that you have put off for many years now. Especially at first, take it easy, and you will get to your desired goal with much less strain and just as quickly. Remember that ease and moderation are the whole idea of this exercise program, and any attempt at overexertion will defeat the purpose.

Let me remind you of a story you have told to yourself many times. Maybe you will have told it a bit differently, but you will recognize it just the same. You are a man of common means, about 40 years old. If you had saved only five dollars a week since you began working, at around 20, do you know how much you would have saved by now? Over $5,000!! You wish now that you had that much saved, don't you? But a measly five dollars a week, only twenty bucks a month, that's not enough to even bother with. It increases too slowly. We have our eyes set on bigger things. And, of course, it's good to set our sights high, to shoot after the finer things in life. But......and I almost hesitate to ask the question......do you have the $5,000? Of course, in reality it would be almost double that amount counting interest, which by now would add more to your total each year than the principal five dollar per week investment.

A STEADY PLAN IS BEST

The point is obvious. You have invested in your future slowly, and easily, but it's paying off handsomely. Few of us have done as well with our big plans and crash programs. But what is more important is the basic underlying principle of SURETY. Maybe the big stock deal came through and maybe it didn't. Maybe the business venture you were planning paid off and maybe it didn't. Maybe you even lost money on both and took a long time to recoup the loses. But regardless of each individual outcome, this true fact remains:

A STEADY, PLANNED PROGRAM IS USUALLY THE BEST WAY TO ACHIEVE A DESIRED GOAL

IT'S YOU I'M WORRIED ABOUT

Rest assured at this point that it is not the difficulty of the exercises that prompts me to sound the caution against overexertion, but rather my fear of your built-in desire to go further just because you feel good. The same way you stay out in the sun too long the first few times and get burned because it doesn't appear to you that you're even getting pink. Let me give you another example.

The Royal Canadian Air Force plan for physical fitness is one of the finest plans I know. It begins at a very low level and works up to where even an accomplished athlete is hard pressed to complete the exercises. I was an instructor in one of the first courses to use this fine plan when it was introduced into the U. S. Air Force in 1962. The groups I was working with were young officers ranging in age from 24 to 30 and in varying degrees of physical fitness. We required them to begin slowly and work up to the more difficult levels, which was the sensible thing to do. But many of them felt the lower levels were too easy and either skipped them or ran through five or six levels in a single day. Soon the effects of this poor start began to show up on some of the men. The exercises got too hard too fast, and their muscles balked at the treatment. We were used to getting many casualties in our competitive athletic program, but this was the first experience we had encountered of casualties in a program of straight exercise. I would like to say it taught the violators a lesson, but it didn't. Its major effect was to sour them on any exercise program, and I suppose that even today they feel they are better off doing without.

Another interesting note. After five years the U. S. Air Force is now in the process of replacing the RCAF program for the very reason that prompted me to write this book: it's too hard, so no one is doing it!

DON'T PRESS YOURSELF

Remember, you're not trying to be an athlete, or to complete this program in any certain length of time. So don't press yourself. If you feel you can do more than you are doing, that's fine, but keep doing just that much for another week or two before you even consider moving up. If you always do a bit less than you can, you will always stay happy in the program. And remember, that's the MAIN thing.

CAREFUL SELECTION

I have selected your exercises very carefully. They are not hard, but at the same time they are effective. There are six of them, and they are arranged to help you do two things:

(1) Start each day gradually
(2) Transition into the exercise that follows

Let me explain what I mean.

Start each day gradually: When you get up in the morning your muscles are stiff from several hours of complete inactivity. The joints are rusty and will crack a little the first few times you move them. After you wash the sleep from your eyes you begin to feel a little better but you still do not feel like doing exercises. The first two exercises on our list, knee lift and side nip-in, are designed just for that feeling. They will limber you and take that tight feeling away. You won't believe this until you try it, but they actually make you feel like you want to do more.

Transition into the exercise that follows: Each of our six exercises sets up our muscles to prepare for the one to follow; thus, no possibility of straining a cold muscle. For this reason it's important that we do them in the order in which they are listed. You will need your book to guide you the first week or so, but soon you will have them memorized and they will come quite naturally to you.

TWO SPECIFIC CAUTIONS

We are only going to do ten repetitions of the first four exercises, and you will see after you have done them for a while that you could scarcely hurt yourself if you wanted to. They are "warmer-uppers" and "stretchers" for the most part, and transition so well that they prevent any likelihood of overexertion for you. But that's not the case with the fifth and sixth exercises, partial push-up, and running-in-place. I list five repetitions of the partial push-up and don't feel you should exceed that number until you're well on your way into the program. In fact, if you have not exercised in years, or if you are grossly over-weight, I would suggest starting with two or three and working your way up to five. Your arms and chest will tell you if you need more work. On the sixth exercise, running-in-place, I recommend doing half the suggested number (100) for at least the first week until you build up your wind a little. At any time follow this rule:

IF YOU ARE OVEREXERTING
SLOW DOWN OR STOP

Then, the next day, start slower and easier.

YOUR SIX EXERCISES

That brings us up to the listing of your exercises. Here they are:

1. Knee lift	10 Repetitions
2. Side nip-in	10 Repetitions
3. Stretcher	10 Repetitions
4. Partial sit-up	10 Repetitions
5. Partial push-up	5 Repetitions
6. Running-in-place	200 Repetitions

I will explain how to do them in chapter six. But first, I would like to discuss another important point with you—will-power.

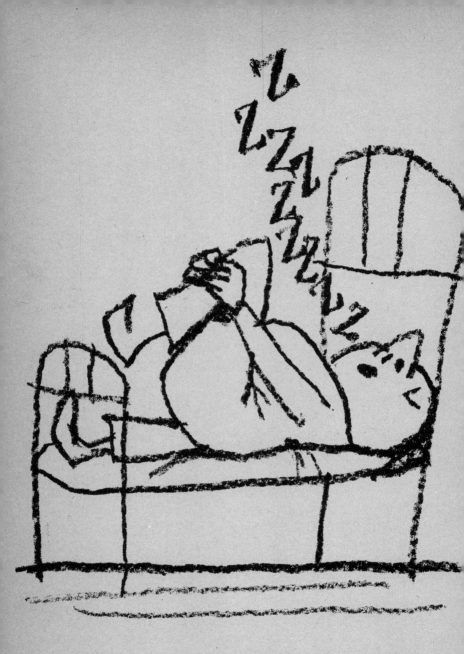

Chapter 5

A WORD ABOUT WILL-POWER

DEVELOPING HABITS

Man is surely a creature of habit. We eat, work, and sleep in substantially the same manner each day and loathe the force that makes us change. We have all noted with humor the small mannerisms that bring this fact to our attention. For a couple of months I used tooth powder on my brush to brush my teeth. I would pour the powder in my hand and pick it up onto the wet brush. After I switched back to toothpaste again I still found myself washing the non-existent powder off my hand when I was through brushing. Have you ever seen the driver of a car use his automobile lighter to light his cigarette, then roll down his window a few inches, shake the lighter to put out the flame, and start to throw it out of the car? Which side of the bed to you sleep on? Which side do you get up on? Which shoe goes on first, which leg in your trousers, which arm in your coat? They're all done by habit.

MOST HABITS ARE GOOD

Sometimes we tend to think that all habits are bad, because those are the ones we hear the most about: smoking, drinking, eating, gossip. But that isn't the case at all. Most habits are good. Indeed, it would be impossible for us to get through the day without relying on habits. Driving our car is at least 50% habit. So is dressing, shaving, showering, eating, walking, and sometimes thinking. Because we all have habits, both good and bad, it becomes our task to learn to live with them. We try to minimize the bad ones, and strengthen the good ones.

But sometimes it's not a matter of merely strengthening a weak habit; we have to create the act first, then create the habit. That's what we want to do with this exercise program. And that's where will-power comes in.

HELP CREATE GOOD HABITS

Habits are created because we get used to doing something without consciously thinking about it. Like our foot automatically going for the brake pedal when we see a stop sign. It didn't do that when we first began driving; we had to think each action through and react directly from thought response. But the habitual response developed quickly because we did the same thing every time. We *always* did the same thing, we had no choice in the matter. If we didn't do it the car simply would not stop and we would be in trouble. The decision was not really in our hands. But if we do have the choice of the decision, as in whether to exercise or not, it takes strong will-power to get us up to the point where our habit will start to help us.

WILL-POWER AND HABITS

That's why I would like you to do these exercises at the same time every day, and in the same place. That's why I would like you to associate doing them with another necessary act that you already do every day, like shave or shower. If you make it a definite point to do them either just before shaving, or just after, or just before showering, habitual help will soon be on its way, and most of the burden will be lifted from you.

I think I should point out again, because I keep talking about the male habits, and his point of view, that these exercises are just as applicable to the female as to

32

the male, and will do just as much good. My main purpose in directing most of my information toward the male is that this plan is actually tailor-made for him because of his limited time, and less specific exercise goals. Females usually have more time that they can afford to spend on an exercise program and, indeed, more time is required if one wishes to gain specific goals such as trimming waist, legs, neck, and increasing the firmness of one's bustline. But this program is also ideal for working girls.

The point on will-power is this:

(1) Give yourself a goal and promise yourself you will not miss a day during that period.
(2) Strongly resist any attemp to miss the first day!

If you feel especially tired and have an overpowering desire to miss a day, just skip *part* of the six exercises. Forget about running-in-place that day and call it a bonus from me. Or skip the partial push-ups, too. No conscience involved on your part—I said you could do it. BUT DO *SOME* OF THE EXERCISES EVERY DAY AT THE SAME TIME YOU USUALLY DO THEM.

By receiving the bonus of a small rest, while still not giving in to the urge to skip a day altogether, you will come back tomorrow refreshed and anxious to keep your good work going.

IDENTIFYING THE DANGER PERIOD

Let me caution you about the time when your WILL-POWER must be at its best:

FROM THE THIRD TO THE SIXTH WEEK !!!

Your beginning initiative, and the newness of the task, will carry you for the first few weeks. You will also be rewarded by many identifiable signs of fitness improvement during this period which will buoy your spirit. But you will get a feeling, sometime after the first few weeks, that the program has ceased to do you much good, and you will suddenly realize that it is becoming more difficult to get yourself to do it. That's the DANGER period—beware of it. It's just the time between the dimming of the early initiative and the blooming of the habit response. It invariably happens, and it's nothing to get concerned about. Smile at it when it comes, because you recognize it, and press on past it.

Remember, these exercises haven't stopped their effectiveness just because you *can't feel them* increasing the fitness of your body. That's precisely the time we're working for, when the exercises have increased the fitness of your body, and because of it have become surprisingly EASY to do.

With those cautions I'll leave the WILL-POWER in your hands.

Chapter 6

THE BASIC PROGRAM

Before we launch into our exercise program let's take a few minutes to examine the exercises, individually and as a group, to see what they are going to do for us.

Here they are listed again, along with the repetitions and the time it takes to do each one:

1.	Knee lift	10 Rep.	:20 Sec.
2.	Side rip-in	10 Rep.	:30 Sec.
3.	Stretcher	10 Rep.	:40 Sec.
4.	Partial sit-up	10 Rep.	:25 Sec.
5.	Partial push-up	5 Rep.	:15 Sec.
6.	Running-in-place	200 Rep.	2:15 Min/Sec.

If you add up the times you will see that it takes about four and one-half minutes to complete the total set, but I will talk more about time later in this chapter. First, let's look at each individual exercise.

KNEE LIFT

This is a very simple exercise (see illustrations in this chapter) that is designed to loosen most of the muscles in your body. Assume the position of this exercise and see for yourself how many muscles and joints are affected.

As you balance on one foot you are automatically limbering the joints of that ankle and knee. Now as you pull your leg up toward your chest, stop and feel what muscles are in play. You can feel the calf and thigh muscle of the leg being pulled, plus the joint of that leg. You can feel the pull on the buttocks of the leg being pulled and upon the thigh of the leg standing. Now let your attention fall on the lower part of your spine and feel the action there. And, of course, the upper portions of your shoulders and spine where the direct effect of your arms pulling against the leg are felt. The limbering-pulling process is reversed when the other leg comes up.

SIDE NIP-IN

This one is partly designed as a loosener but also incorporates a beneficial body-shaping action. It will help slim your waist and improve the tightness of your midsection, which will help any of your reaching and stretching motions. This exercise, although simple to do, can take inches off your waistline over a period of a few months. The more vigorous the action of the nip-in, the more beneficial the effect on your waist. You will also note that the lower spine and legs take an active part in this exercise. It is very similar to the action that a good golfer takes when he puts his hips and legs through a golf shot.

STRETCHER

With the stretcher we begin to get a little more serious about exercise. The first two exercises do not really incorporate large enough displacement of our body to involve wind or endurance. After a couple of weeks you will find that there is really no limit to the number of them you can do. But exercise three, the stretcher, does displace a large volume of our body weight, and thus it does require endurance. It is one of the best exercises we can do because it involves so much of our body. If I had to choose one single immobile exercise with which to stay fit, not being allowed to use any other, I would choose this stretcher. There is very little of the body that this one doesn't reach. Take the position and see for yourself. The first thing you will feel is the pull on the long muscle on the back of your legs, trying to stop you from bending down all the way, and the strong muscle of your calf which will harden as you do. Then you will note the stretching on your midsection, your spine, your shoulders, your back, your arms, practically your whole body. As you come up and bend the upper part of your body backwards you will realign your spine naturally between your shoulder blades, and spread out and flex your chest and shoulder muscles. You don't have to keep your knees stiff when you do this exercise. Let them bend a bit if they want. It will get easier as you progress and soon your hands will make the floor with hardly any bend in the knees at all. Suit it to yourself; you will be able to tell how far you can easily stretch. This is one exercise that you will never get completely used to. Every morning regardless of how long you have done it, you will feel the stretching in your legs for the first few repetitions. But you won't encounter any difficulty picking up the newspaper any more!

PARTIAL SIT-UP

This is the only one in which you might have problems—I don't know how large your bathroom is. If there isn't enough room to stretch full length on the floor, you may pull up your knees and complete the exercise in exactly the same manner as if your legs were straight. We all know what effect the sit-up has on our body; it's a stomach flattener and tightener. It also exercises the neck and shoulders. The partial sit-up does the same thing, only not quite so harshly.

PARTIAL PUSH-UP

The partial push-up is another exerciser and conditioner. At first it may leave you a trifle breathless. As I mentioned earlier, do only two or three to begin with if you find you are having trouble making the whole five. This partial push-up will strengthen your arms, chest, and shoulders practically as well as any exercise can. You are weight lifting in a sense. You are lifting your body weight the distance of the length of your arms. Naturally a very heavy person will not be able to do this as easily as a not-so-heavy one. Don't fret. As your arms and chest grow stronger and your endurance increases, you'll be surprised how easy it becomes. A word of caution: the edge of your bathtub may be slippery; make sure you have a good hold throughout this exercise. Most home accidents occur in the kitchen, and we don't want to be responsible for changing that trend.

RUNNING-IN-PLACE

Running is the best and most natural conditioner of them all. Its effect reaches every part of our body as a conditioner, and does a good job of exercising much of the rest. Running, and its use of the internal organs, is especially beneficial as a means of counteracting those bad habits of ours, smoking, drinking, and unwise eating. It seems to reach deep down into our system and flush out the carbon of inactivity and over indulgence. Actually it just acts as a tune-up to our organs and circulation system so that they do the job for us. One thing running does do that most doctors agree upon is build up the capacity of our lungs, and strengthen and develop the blood vessels in our muscles and heart. This means that our lungs have a greater capacity for work and play, and that our heart does less work in completing its job of continually supplying our body with blood. The results of those body functions can only lead to better health and a physically more fruitful life. I spoke earlier of limiting this exercise to half the given number of repetitions until you've completed at least the first week. I'll say it again. Don't overexert yourself. If your lungs begin to burn, slow down or stop. It will not hurt you, but it is unnecessary as we are in no hurry to get to any set point. USE GOOD JUDGMENT.

THEY GO TOGETHER

There they are, all six of them Each. one, you have noted, is designed to do a specific function. You will find that they blend harmoniously together, smoothly working in to each other to arrive at our overall goal. The knee lift loosens our muscles and sets our body in the proper environment; the side nip-in continues the warm-up while exercising the waist and legs; the stretcher completes the warm-up while at the same time exercising many muscles and beginning our endurance conditioning; the partial sit-up strengthens stomach, and upper torso; the partial push-up strengthens arms, chest, and shoulders; running-in-place strengthens legs, lungs, heart, and rounds out the condition of every part of our body.

I hope you see that although it is simple, and takes only five minutes of our time, it is thorough and deals with every function of our body that we use in everyday pursuits.

ABOUT TIME

The preface of this book promises that you can become fit on only five minutes a day. And I think you can see now that it can be done. I have timed the exercises dozens of times to come up with the times I listed earlier in this chapter. These times, which total four minutes and 25 seconds, represent the recommended speed at which these exercises should be done. Therefore, it would be well for you to time yourself the first few days until you begin to have a feel for the proper cadence. You may go immediately from one exercise right on to the next except in two instances. I would recommend a 15-second or so rest after the stretcher and after the partial push-up.

Remember this point:

TIME IS RELATIVE

That this exercise program takes only five minutes to complete is not its major value. Its value is that it can give you a well-rounded exercise program that will be USEFUL to you, in just five minutes. Anything else, although it wouldn't take much time, would be a waste of the time it did take. I'm sure the thought has crossed your mind that it takes a good runner less than four minutes to run a mile. But what he does in that four minutes would surely kill most of us off, wouldn't it? The time spent doing that would not only be wasted, but harmful. My concern has been to put together a program that will make you, an AVERAGE person, into a happier, healthier, and more useful one; and to do it in the amount of time that you will be willing to give.

The exercises follow.

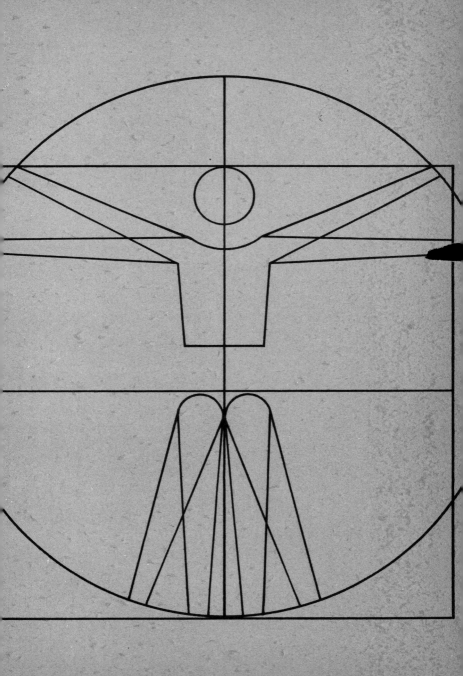

Exercise 1

Knee Lift

---

10 Repetitions
20 Seconds

This exercise is done in two counts. Standing upright, bring the right leg upward toward the chest, bending it at the knee. In the same motion grasp with both hands and pull further upward toward chest. Count ONE is made as the arms make their pull, count TWO when the right foot comes back down. Then repeat same procedure with the left leg. Each leg receives five pulls.

FOLLOW-ON EXERCISE: #7

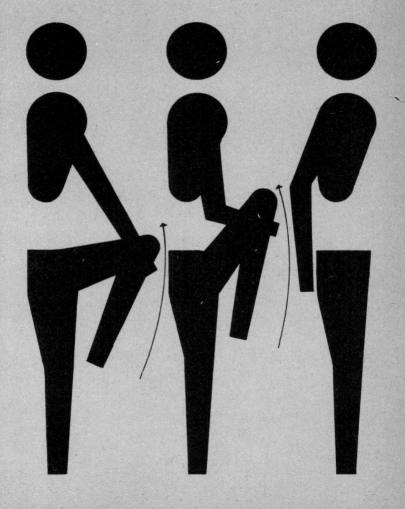

Exercise **2**

Side Nip-In

---

10 Repetitions
30 Seconds

This exercise is done in four counts. Standing upright, widen legs to slightly more than shoulder width, resting hands on hips. Remaining upright, bend to the right, forcing the waist and hips to move to the left. Legs and right knee should also move to the left. Repeat the nip-in movement four times for one repetition, then begin on the left side. Make the movement vigorous enough to feel it thrust in at your waist. Count the ten repetitions this way: 1-2-3-1, 1-2-3-2, 1-2-3-3, 1-2-3-4, 1-2-3-5, etc.

FOLLOW-ON EXERCISE: #8

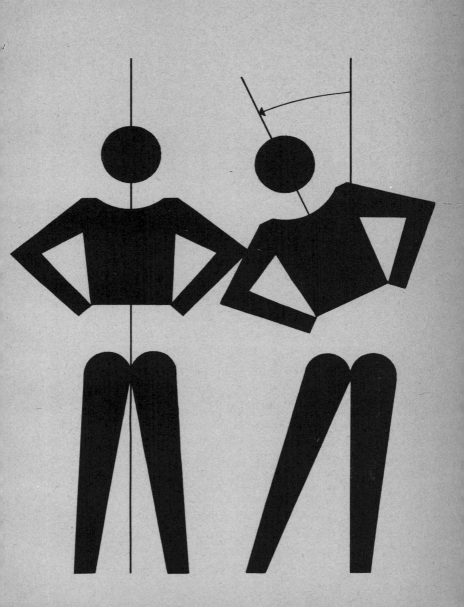

Exercise 3

Stretcher

---

10 Repetitions
40 Seconds

This exercise is also done in four counts. Stand upright, feet spread about 18 inches apart, and place hands on hips for starting position. On count ONE, bend at waist and touch the floor in front of your left foot with your finger tips. On count TWO, bounce up eight inches and touch floor halfway between your legs. On count THREE, bounce up again and touch floor in front of right foot, and on count FOUR come back up and bend backward. Do not strain to keep knees from bending, but make each bounce come about eight inches off floor. On the fourth count, backward bend, come back far enough to feel slight pull in shoulder blades and chest. Count 1-2-3-1, 1-2-3-2, 1-2-3-3, and change direction to move from right foot to left after five repetitions.

FOLLOW-ON EXERCISE: #9

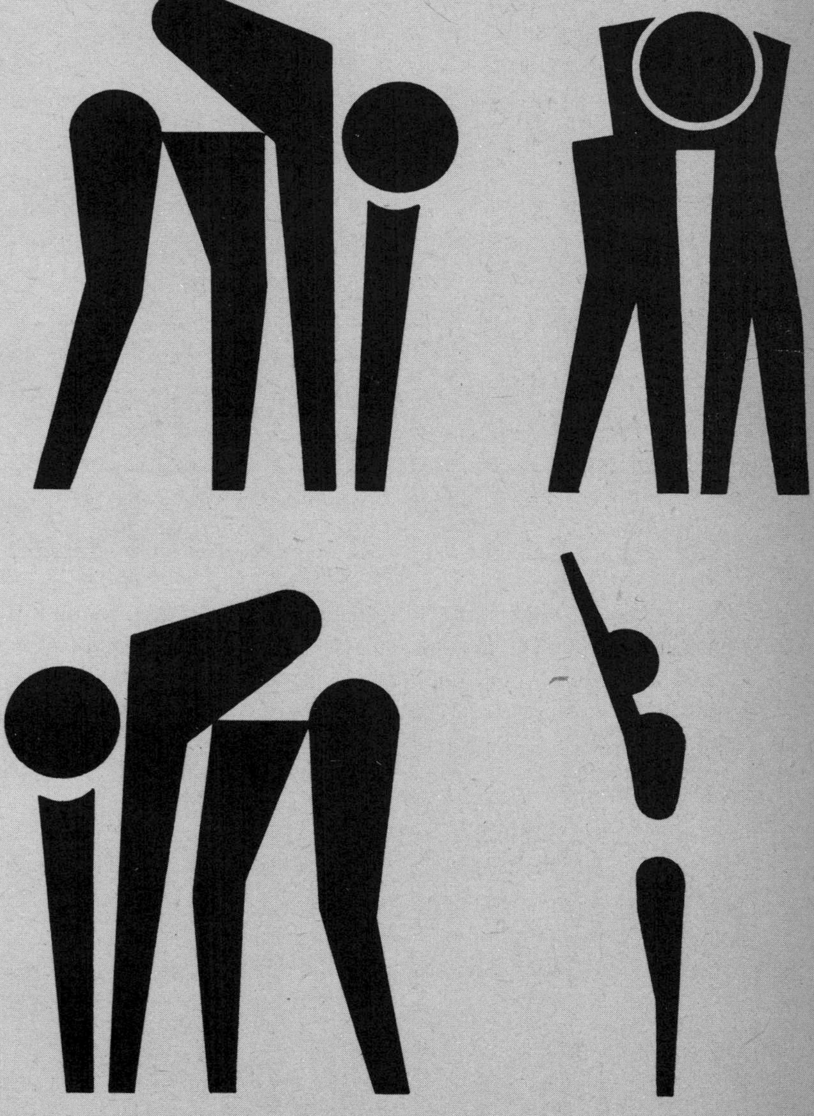

Exercise **4**

Partial Sit-Up

---

10 Repetitions
25 Seconds

Two counts to this exercise. Lie on your back on the floor with your hands along your sides. On count ONE bring head and shoulders off the ground far enough to look at your ankles. Pause slightly, and on count TWO, bring head back down. Head should come up high enough to let you feel the pull in your stomach. If you are doing the exercise with your legs pulled up because of space limitation, come up high enough for your shoulder blades to just clear the floor.

FOLLOW-ON EXERCISE: #10

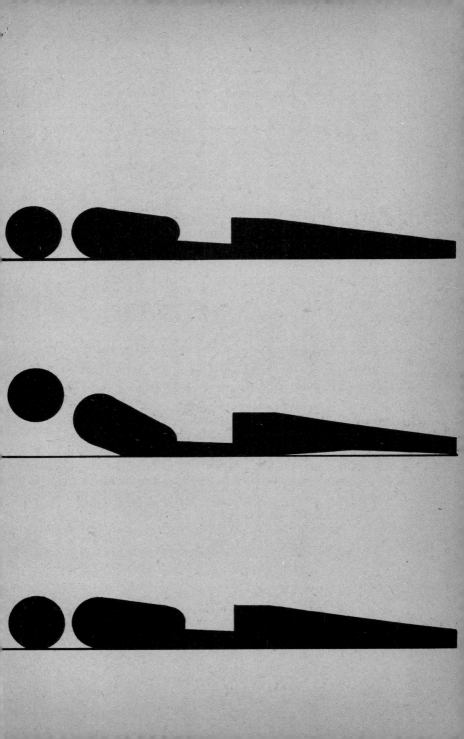

Exercise **5**

Partial Push-Up

---

5 Repetitions
15 Seconds

Place your hands firmly on the side of the bathtub, your arms straight, directly under your shoulders. Slide your feet out to full length so that your arms are supporting most of your weight and only your toes touch the floor. You may have your buttocks elevated slightly for balance if you wish. Lower your chest down toward the tub until it is within a few inches of the surface, and straighten arms back out again for one repetition. Work up to five if you find the first few difficult. Rest a few seconds after completing. BE CAREFUL OF A SLIPPERY TUB!

FOLLOW-ON EXERCISE: #11

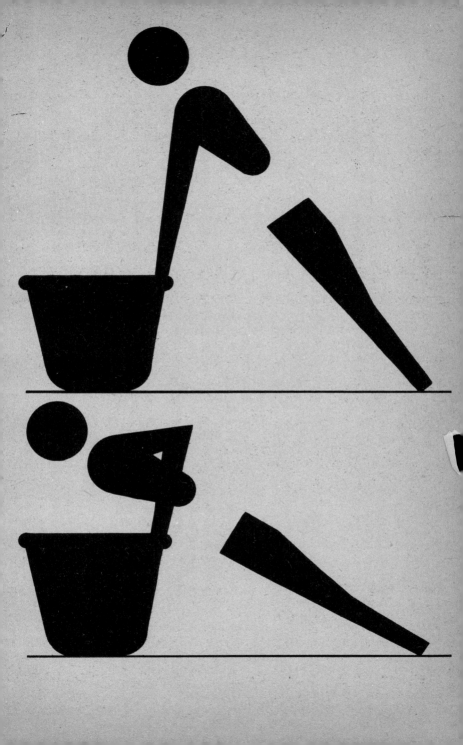

Running-In-Place

---

200 Repetitions
2:15 Min/Sec.

Begin by merely marking time with a left and right beat as though you were marching. Then quicken into a jogging motion, lifting the knees so that the feet come about two inches off the floor. Count one count each time left foot touches the floor. As the run becomes natural you may want to swing your arms just a little for balance. Begin with a hundred repetitions (200 steps) the first week and increase to 200 slowly. If you should desire more of a workout when you feel good, merely bring the knees a bit higher.

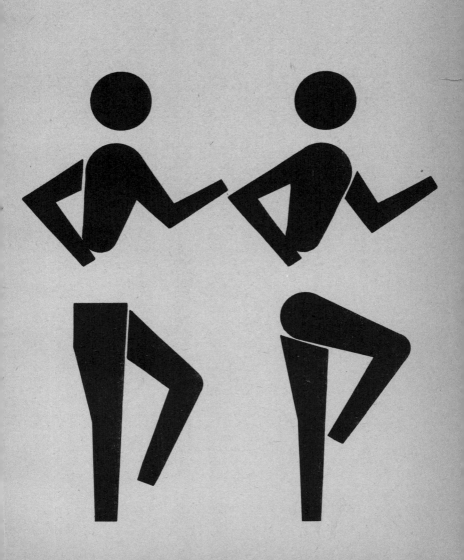

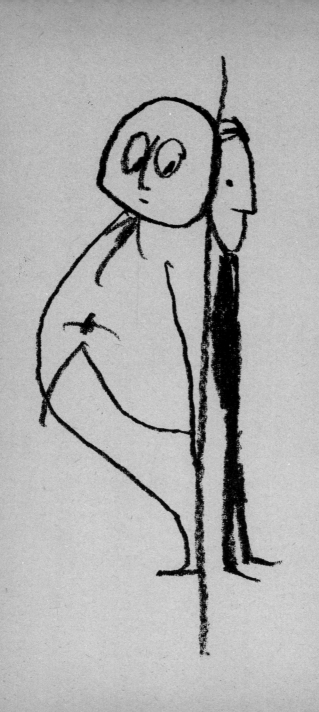

Chapter 7

SOME CHECKS ON YOUR HEALTH

One of the most often discussed "signposts" of health is a person's weight. It is normally considered that if a person is overweight he is less healthy than a person who is not. Of course that is a generalization that may or may not be true. Many overweight people are very healthy, and conversely, many average-weight people are not. But these two points about body weight are true in all cases:

(1) The more body weight a person carries, the more energy it takes to move it around.
(2) The more energy one uses, the harder the heart must work to supply the body with blood.

Thus, an overweight person in normal day-to-day operation will work harder and require more work from his body than a person who is not overweight. I will discuss how much more work the heart does in a moment. Right now let me say a word or two more about your weight.

YOUR "NATURAL" WEIGHT

Each of us has what I will call a "natural weight". It is the weight our body seeks under normal, healthy, conditions. It is the weight our body will return to when it is given the chance to decide for itself. Our "natural" weight is the end result of all we do and think, but basically it is governed by these three factors:

(1) One's natural body structure
(2) One's normal eating habits
(3) One's natural disposition (nervous or sedentary)

Notice that it is a combination of the three factors that decides our natural body weight. If we are normal or average in all three, we are likely to be normal or average in our weight. If any one of the factors becomes stronger than the others, an imbalance will occur. For instance, we have all known the person whose natural disposition is high-strung and nervous. Because of this his activity is not normal, he can't sit still and his body is constantly on the move. As a result he can eat like a horse and never gain a pound. All the food he can take in is immediately needed as fuel to run his over-active body, none of it turning into stored fat or excess weight.

On the other hand our disposition may be sedentary, which means that we must be very careful about our food intake because our naturally inactive body needs only a limited amount to keep it going, and the excess will surely be stored as fat.

DETERMINE YOUR "NATURAL" WEIGHT

I bring up the discussion of "natural" weight because most of us know what our own "natural" weight is. And it may or may not fall within the limits given to us on a weight chart. If you do know your own natural weight, turn to the weight chart in the appendix and check them against one another. If you really don't know your natural weight, I'm sure your family physician can help you determine one very easily.

I think it's important that you know your natural weight and use it as your weight measuring stick rather than a weight picked off a weight chart. I constantly meet people who are worried about being overweight, or underweight, when they actually are not at all. They merely have abnormal body structure, or function, or disposition that is difficult to show on a simple chart. Indeed, just the capacity that each individual body has to retain its liquid can mean several pounds difference in our weight.

YOUR BEATING HEART

Few of us realize it but we have a built-in work recorder in our body, our heart. It will tell you at any time exactly how hard it is working to accomplish its job, and although there are many other factors involved in the operation, the heartbeat is a pretty good indication of our bodies' efficiency.

It can be stated this way:

THE FEWER BEATS IT TAKES THE HEART TO SUPPLY THE BODY WITH BLOOD, THE MORE EFFICIENT THE HEART IS.

Of course, as always, there are other factors that must be considered, such as size and flexibility of blood vessels, and the many impediments of circulation; but in general, a more efficient heart will work less to accomplish a given job.

FEEL IT BEAT

As I sit here writing my pulse rate is 70 beats per minute. I know that I must be quite relaxed for it to be there, for when I take my annual physical examination it is usually between 74 and 78. If I lie down it drops to 66. If I stand up it will be 72. If I get even an anxious thought it will rise quickly, and I can feel the increase as I get the thought. The marvelous communication system of

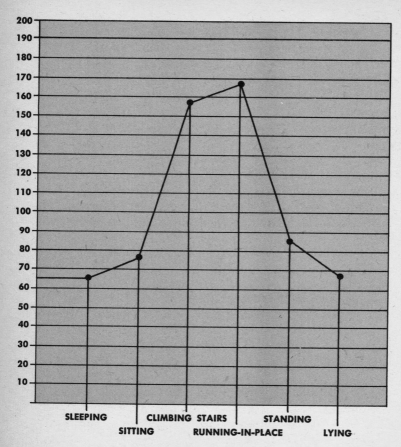

SLEEPING		CLIMBING STAIRS		STANDING
	SITTING	RUNNING-IN-PLACE		LYING

Here is a graphic illustration of the number of heart beats it takes an average person to accomplish different daily tasks. Running-in-place has been included as a comparison against your common routine.

the body is telling the heart that something important or strenuous is about to happen, and our body will require more blood and oxygen to the muscles to cope with it. Look at the chart on this page and see how the pulse rate of the heart can be an indication of the work we are doing.

By keeping tabs on your pulse rate you can tell if the fitness efforts you are making are paying dividends in physical efficiency. For instance: take your pulse now for one minute and note the count. Multiply that number by 60 to get your hourly count. And again by 24 for your daily total. Your answer probably falls somewhere between 140,000 and 200,000 beats for a 24-hour period. As you increase your fitness, watch your daily total drop. If you are now at 200,000 and in four weeks under the same conditions your heart is pumping only 170,000 times, you have saved your heart 30,000 beats of needless work each day.

For fun, check your rate while you're doing your exercises too. And again after you're through. It will help you progress and will help you chart your own fitness. On the run-in-place try to keep the speed of the run sufficient to make you just a trifle short of breath. You won't have any trouble doing this at first, but later on you will. It usually takes about 120 beats or so per minute to cause breath shortage, but check yourself and see what your own level is. But remember that it will be coming down steadily, so adjust. When your usual running rate is not producing a slight shortness of breath by the end of the run, either increase the speed of the steps, or the height your feet come off the ground. Either one displaces more weight and causes more energy to be expended.

Use both the "natural weight" check and the pulse rate check to your advantage.

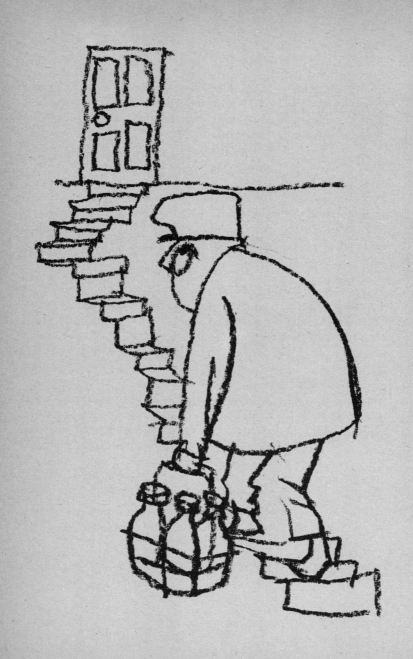

Chapter 8

TAILORING THE PROGRAM TO YOU

Some of you may think that you do not fall into the general grouping of individuals who will obtain the most benefit from a "set" program of exercises. You may be right, although your circumstances would have to be quite unusual.

If you work as a milkman in an area where the apartment buildings don't have elevators, I would guess that your legs are already in pretty good shape from your daily workout on the stairs. You may want to substitute another exercise for the knee lift.

If you work as a musician, playing trumpet in a band your stomach is already strong from the workout you give it blowing your horn regularly. You may want to substitute another exercise for the partial sit-up; one that is more vigorous and would do you more good.

Then too, there will be a few of you who will have a desire to go on to more difficult exercises when these become too easy for you. I again caution this group against over-enthusiasm. If you progress to the point that your exercises become a burden to you, the temptation to discontinue will be greater and you will lose more than you will gain. Slow and steady is still BEST.

ADDITIONAL EXERCISES

But for all of you, I have included in the appendix additional exercises that can be incorporated into your daily schedule, either as a substitute or as a more advanced "follow-on" to the basic program. Here's how to use it: you will notice that on each explanation page of the basic program there is an addition at the bottom reading FOLLOW-ON, followed by a number. That FO number is the number of the exercise in the appendix that is the natural follow-on of the exercise on that page. For instance, in the case of the milkman who feels he needs a stronger exercise than #1, the knee lift, he can see that the follow-on number is #7, which, turning to the appendix exercises, is the deep knee bend. He may substitute. The trumpet player will find that the follow-on to the partial sit-up is exercise #10, the full sit up. He may substitute.

If any of you really have the desire to advance to more difficult exercises you can easily advance the entire program by merely adding six to the number of the exercise listed in the basic program. Thus, appendix exercises #7, #8, #9, #10, and #11 are the follow-ons for the first five exercises of the basic program. Merely add the running-in-place to them, also increased in repetitions if you like, and you have upgraded the entire set.

Also, an additional eight exercises are included in the appendix for those with special exercise goals.

A WORD OF WISDOM

Just as each of us is aware of our own "natural" weight, we also are privately aware of our own worst indulgences. We live with our own bodies constantly and we get to know them pretty well. We know especially when they are feeling bad, and usually what caused the condition. Some of us can't eat pizza without paying the price of indigestion. For others it is something else. We also are aware of the three main indulgences that I spoke of earlier, over-eating, drinking, and smoking, and how our own body reacts to each of them. Let me talk about each for just a moment.

Over-Eating

This is undoubtedly the most common weakness of all. Most of us are plagued by it soon after the activity of youth ceases to burn away the additional food that we take in. The temptations are constantly before us, and therefore we have to take constant care to overcome them. Most of us just try to strike a happy medium, which isn't a bad idea. If over-eating is your problem, this exercise program will help you in these ways: (1) the stretcher will help eliminate that stuffed feeling; (2) the stretcher, side nip-in, and partial sit-up will trim your midsection and strengthen the body tone; (3) the running will put spring in your walk and lighten your weight load.

Drinking

Too much drinking has somewhat the same effect on our bodies that over-eating does, but it carries another threat. We do our drinking IN ADDITION to eating and therefore the caloric intake is especially critical. Alcohol is a concentrated sugar and is charged with more calories than most of us realize (a single martini is 135 calories). Then too, the social acceptance of drinking, as well as its physical effect on our system, create an added desire to over-indulge. Like eating, it would be well for us to cut down; but either way, this exercise program will benefit the drinker in these ways: (1) give the body a physical stimulation each day to improve circulation and blood flow; (2) combat mental fatigue which may have its outlet in the unnecessary drink; and (3) give the body a stronger foundation with which to bounce back to normality after being consecutively stimulated and depressed by too much alcohol.

Smoking

There is today wide controversy over the effects of too much smoking. Generally, most doctors agree that we can considerably cut the harmful effects of smoking by not smoking too much. Moderate smoking has disproportionately less telling effect on the health of the body than does higher consumption. Conversely, high consumption gives proportionately higher chances for harmful effects. Exercise probably can do more to combat the effects of smoking than anything else, short of cutting down or quitting, that we can do. Cigarette smoking as a direct cause of disease or illness is currently undergoing the scrutiny of intense medical research, but all signs point toward controls which will inform the public of its danger. Right now the larger danger lies in the irritation that smoking can cause to an already weak or unhealthy body. By building up the fitness of our body through this exercise program we will not only benefit from the health that is indiscernible to the average person, but we will be able to recognize a considerable improvement in our tolerance to smoking through the realization of (1) better wind, (2) less lung and throat congestion, and (3) stronger endurance.

Appendix

Desirable

MEN

	20 YEARS OLD				30 YEARS OLD & OLDER			
HEIGHT* Feet Inches		SMALL FRAME	MEDIUM FRAME	LARGE FRAME	HEIGHT* Feet Inches		SMALL FRAME	MEDIUM FRAME	LARGE FRAME
5	0	103	114	128	5	0	111	123	138
5	1	105	117	131	5	1	113	125	140
5	2	108	120	135	5	2	115	128	144
5	3	111	123	138	5	3	118	131	147
5	4	114	127	143	5	4	122	135	152
5	5	118	131	147	5	5	125	139	156
5	6	122	135	152	5	6	129	143	161
5	7	125	139	156	5	7	132	147	165
5	8	129	143	161	5	8	136	151	170
5	9	132	147	165	5	9	141	156	175
5	10	136	151	170	5	10	145	161	181
5	11	141	156	175	5	11	150	167	188
6	0	145	161	181	6	0	156	173	194
6	1	150	166	186	6	1	161	179	202
6	2	154	171	192	6	2	167	185	208
6	3	159	176	198	6	3	172	191	215
6	4	164	181	204	6	4	177	197	222

*Without shoes or clothing

Weight Chart

WOMEN

20 YEARS OLD				30 YEARS OLD & OLDER			
HEIGHT* Feet Inches		SMALL FRAME	MEDIUM FRAME	LARGE FRAME	HEIGHT* Feet Inches		SMALL FRAME	MEDIUM FRAME	LARGE FRAME
4	9	96	107	119	4	9	102	113	127
4	10	98	109	123	4	10	104	115	129
4	11	100	111	125	4	11	105	117	132
5	0	103	114	128	5	0	107	119	134
5	1	105	117	132	5	1	110	122	137
5	2	108	120	135	5	2	113	125	141
5	3	111	123	138	5	3	116	129	145
5	4	113	126	142	5	4	119	132	149
5	5	117	130	146	5	5	123	136	153
5	6	121	134	151	5	6	126	140	158
5	7	124	138	155	5	7	130	144	162
5	8	127	141	159	5	8	133	148	167
5	9	131	145	163	5	9	136	151	170
5	10	134	149	168	5	10	140	155	174
5	11	139	154	173	5	11	143	159	179
6	0	144	159	178	6	0	147	164	184

*Without shoes or clothing

Follow-on Exercises

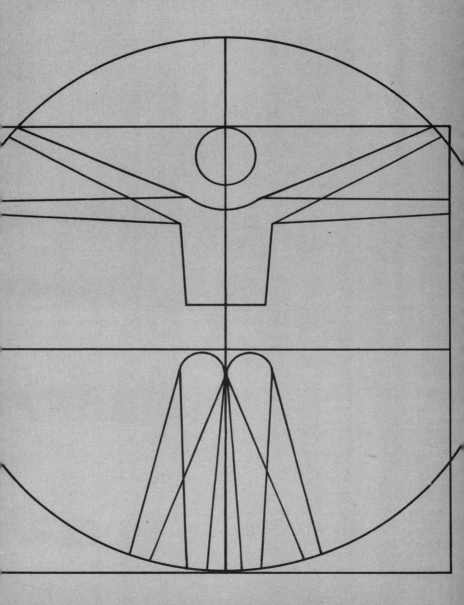

Deep Knee Bends

This exercise is designed to strengthen the muscles and joints in the legs. It is especially good for the knees. Do the exercise in four counts. On count ONE, bend the knees and go halfway down. On count TWO, go all the way. Count THREE, come halfway up and pause. Count FOUR, come back up to the starting position. Do not attempt to do this exercise until you are sure that your knees and legs are already in fairly good shape, otherwise an undue strain will be put on the knee joints. Ten repetitions is sufficient even in an advanced program.

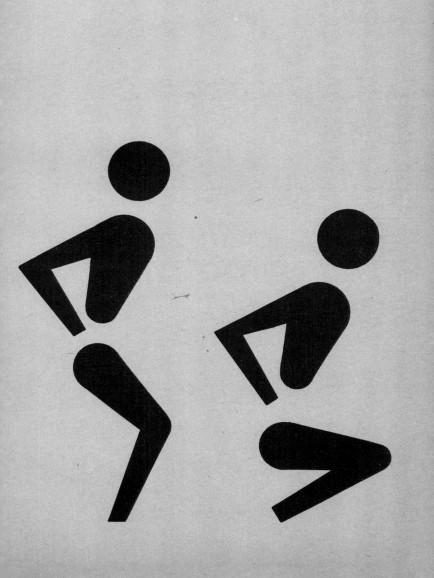

Trunk Rotation

This exercise is used mainly as a conditioner for the midsection. It is similar to the side nip-in except that it rotates in all four directions rather than just left and right. Begin in the upright position with hands on hips and do the exercise in four counts. Count ONE, nip-in to the left, count TWO, nip-in to the front by putting your head and shoulders to the front. On count THREE, nip-in on the right, and on count FOUR, return to starting position, bending slightly backward as you do. This exercise may be done as many as 20 repetitions and is best when used before more difficult exercises. To prevent dizziness, reverse direction after half your repetitions.

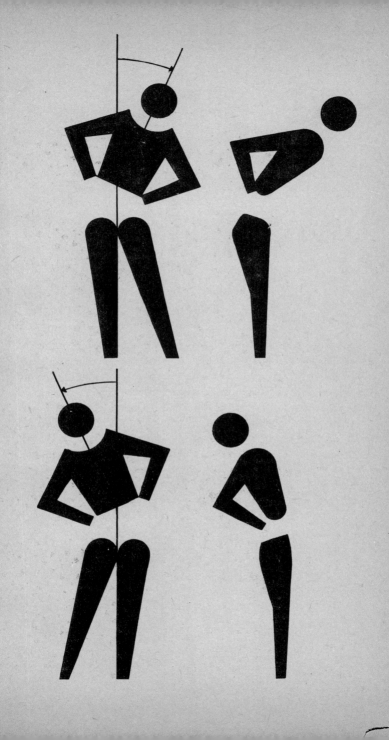

Bouncer

Do this exercise in four counts. Starting position is with legs spread far apart, about twice shoulder width, hands on hips. On count ONE, bend forward and touch hands to floor directly in front of you. On count TWO, bounce up eight inches and touch floor in line with heels of your feet. On count THREE, bounce eight inches and touch floor as far back between your legs as you can reach (if you can't hit floor on third count merely aim at floor and stretch far back). Count FOUR, come back to starting position with slight backward bend. This exercise stretches the legs, arms, shoulders, and back. It should not be used until your body has been conditioned to the pulling and stretching required by it.

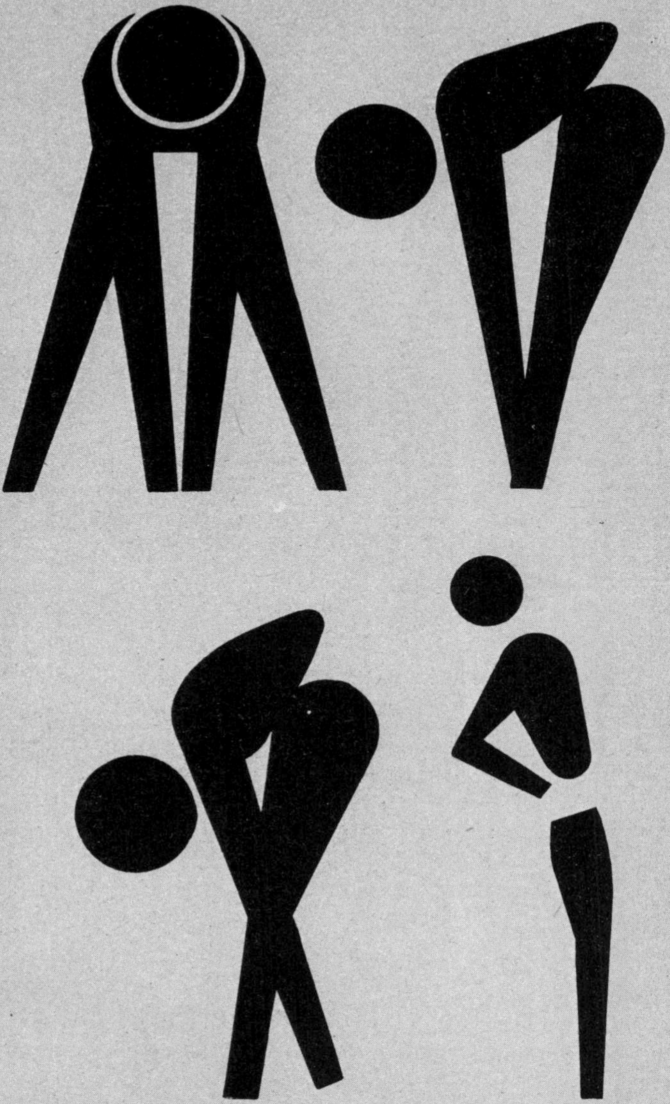

Sit-Up

This is one of the best for tightening and strengthening stomach muscles. Lie full length on back with arms outstretched. You may want to place feet under a chair to hold them down but that is not necessary. Lift the upper part of your body up by pulling from your stomach and shoulders. Come up far enough to touch fingertips to toes. Then return to starting position to complete one repetition. If legs come up or if knees bend just let them. Twenty-five or thirty repetitions is plenty for this exercise. Work up to that number slowly in order to prevent stomach stiffness and soreness.

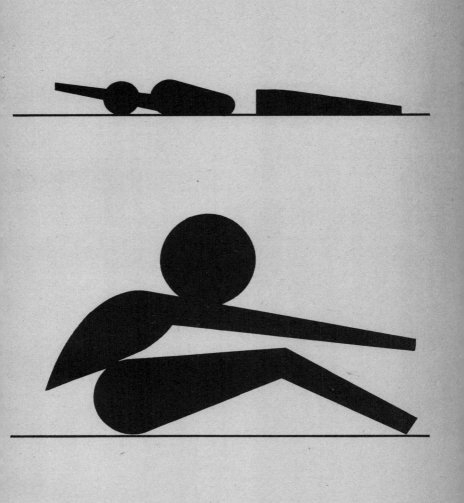

Exescise **11**

Push-Up

This exercise has always been associated with masculine body-building and endurance. Lie full length on stomach, placing hands at shoulder width near where your shoulder and chest meet. Press up with your arms and hold your body off the floor at arms length with only your hands and toes touching floor. This is the starting position. Now lower body toward the floor until chest is within at least two inches of floor, then push-up and return to starting position for one repetition. This is an excellent all-around strength and endurance builder. Twenty-five or thirty repetitions is plenty for the average man. Women need not attempt this one. Use only partial push-up.

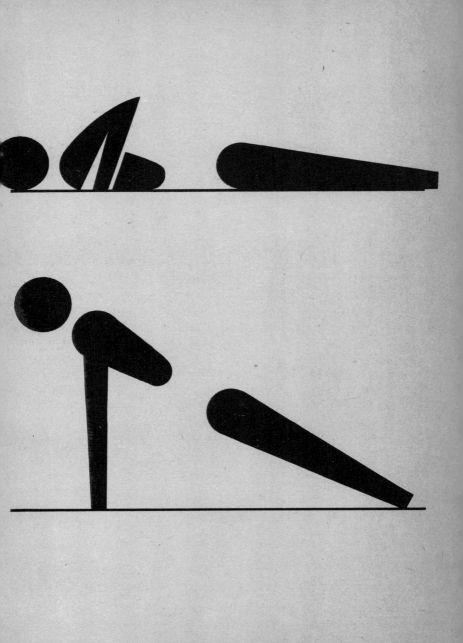

Neck Drill

Here is a good exercise to loosen your neck and upper spine. It will help prevent neck and shoulder fatigue and make you less susceptible to painful neck crick. It is simple: standing upright with hands on hips, bend head to one side, then follow by bending forward, to the opposite side, and to the back. Make about three revolutions going one way, then reverse directions and do another three. When you are finished you may naturally realign your neck and spine by moving your shoulders, arms, and head in a gentle "settling" motion.

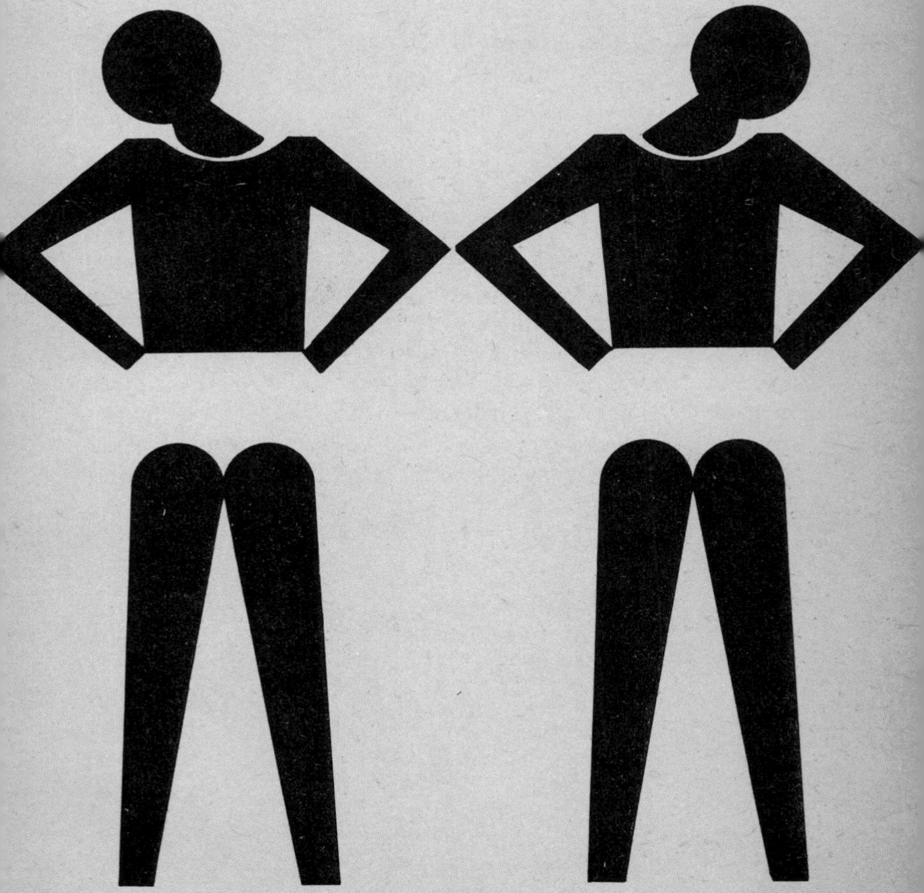

Leg-Lift

The leg-lift is designed to strengthen the muscles of the stomach, chest, and legs. It is not as effective as the sit-up for this purpose but is much easier to accomplish and can actually be done while leaning back in a deep chair. For this exercise, lie full-length on your back with your arms along your sides. Lift the feet up about six inches off the floor and hold them there for about ten seconds. Your head will come up naturally as your stomach muscles tighten to bear the weight of your legs. Repeat three times.

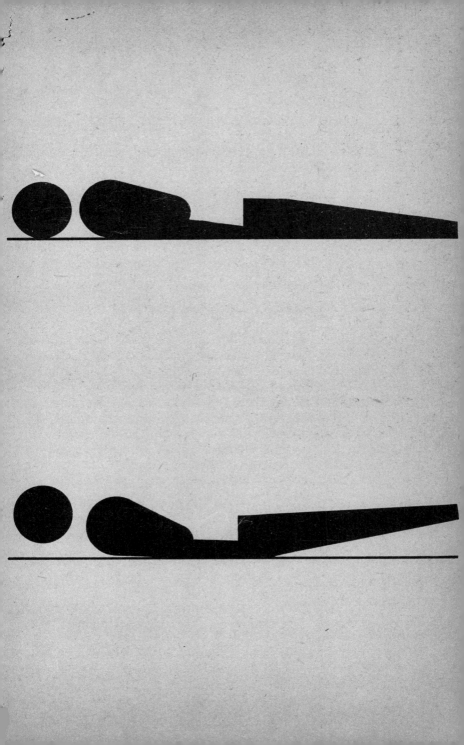

Leg Charger

This exercise is an advanced strengthener for the legs and should not be attempted until you have built a proper foundation for it. It is done in four counts. From a starting position with legs spread wide apart, turn the right foot sideways and lean the body to the far right so that your weight is over your right leg. Use hands lightly for balance. On count ONE press on leg, count TWO bounce up slightly and press again, count THREE another press, and return to starting position on count FOUR. Then repeat the procedure going to the left side.

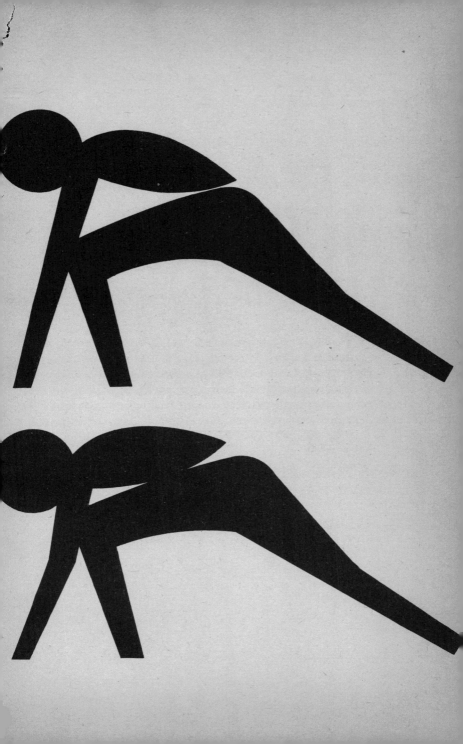

Leg Kicks

This is simply a high kick, similar to the kind chorus girls do every day. It is mainly for the thigh muscles of the leg but also reaches to the stomach and chest. Don't kick too high the first few times you attempt it or you may lose your balance and fall backwards as the weight of the kicking leg may sweep the stationary leg from under you. From an upright standing position gather a slight forward momentum and make a high kick. Reach out the hand of the side you're kicking from as a target to help keep balance. You can add some coordination practice to it later by kicking the opposite side hand with the opposite side foot. Try five with each leg.

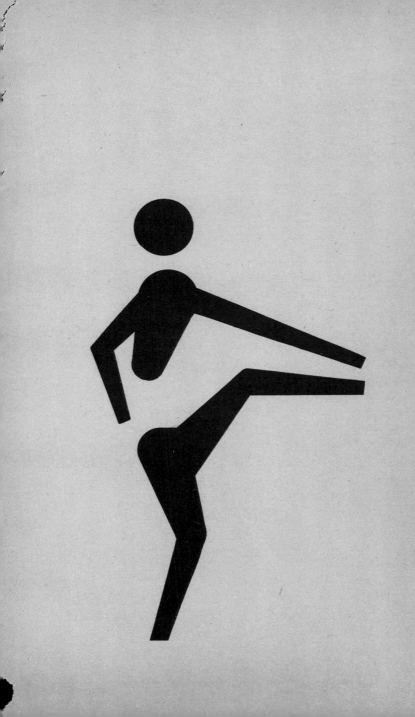

Exercise **16**

Stretch-Up

This is a very good stretcher for the whole body. It is used mainly as a warm-up and can be incorporated into any program. Standing upright with arms in the natural running position, stretch all muscles as high as you can toward the ceiling. Come up on your tiptoes, stretch your stomach, your chest, arms, and even your fingers. Give the legs, stomach, and hands an especially good stretch. Think in your mind that you are actually trying to "throw" yourself to the ceiling. Then come down and repeat the movement again. Do ten repetitions.

Squat Thrust

You likely remember this exercise from your Junior High gym class. It is used mainly for young people because it requires so much active body movement and weight displacement. It is designed to strengthen the arms, chest, back, and legs, and to increase endurance. It is an advanced exercise that you probably won't want to do unless you intend to increase your physical capacity. Begin in the standing position and do it in four counts. On count one drop straight down to the squating position with your palms on the floor. On count two throw your legs to the rear reaching full length and supporting yourself by your arms and toes as in the push-up position, and on the fourth count return to standing. Ten of these is a pretty good work out.

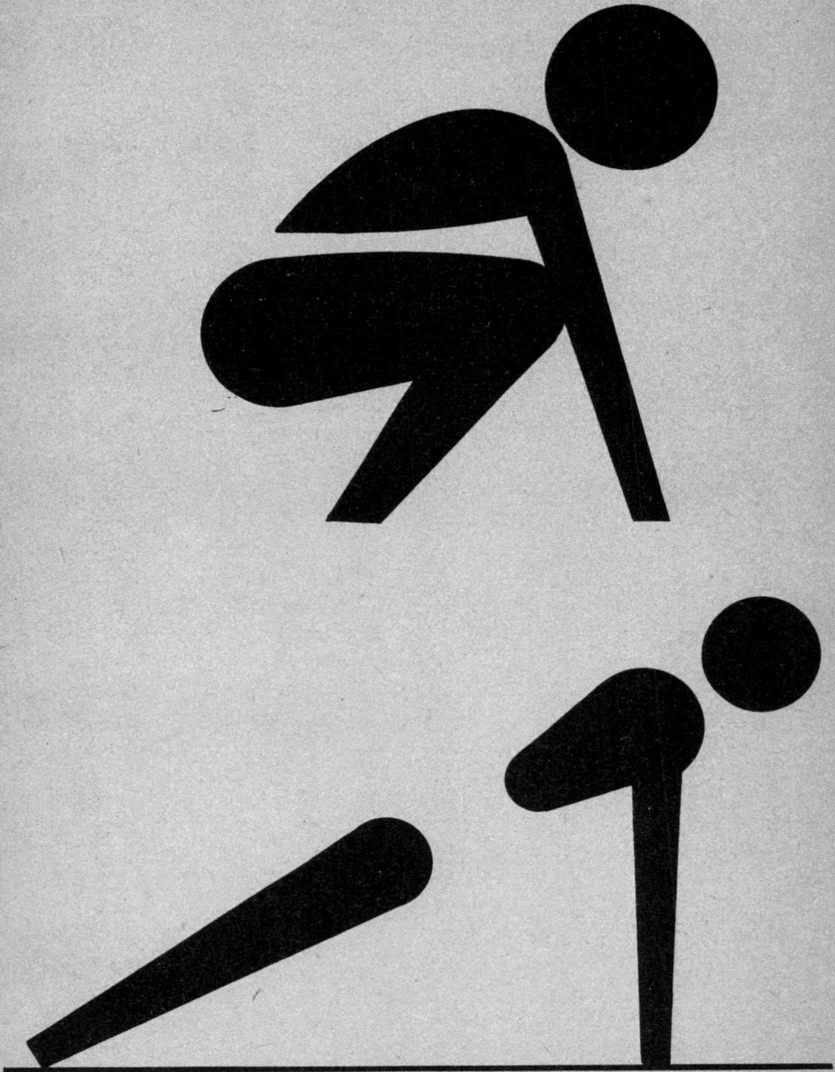

Leg Thrust

The leg thrust is probably the most rigorous conditioner for the legs that you will want to do. It is also a fine endurance strengthener and inner body conditioner and as such should not be attempted until you have already achieved a reasonable degree of physical fitness through less demanding ones. Assume a squat-charge position as you see on the next page with hands spread wide enough apart to balance your weight easily. On each count the legs will change positions in a sort of a charging-in-place motion. It is done in two counts, counting one repetition each time the leg makes the complete cycle. Ten repetitions is plenty.

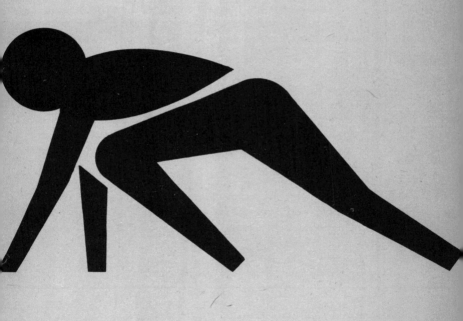

Arm Thrust

This exercise is something like punching a heavy bag only without the bag. It is meant to condition the arms, chest, and shoulders, and to build endurance. This is not a shadow boxing exercise nor is it done in the traditional boxer's stance. Assume a position with the legs spread slightly more than shoulder width apart and lined up evenly (one leg is not advanced as in the boxing stance). Square off your shoulders in the same even position as your legs, with one arm extended horizontal to the floor and the other cocked in the back position. Keep fist square so that the palm would face the floor if you opened it up. On the count of one, throw a vigorous punch with the back arm, at the same time returning the arm that started in front, to the back position. At the count of two, repeat the maneuver. Make each thrust vigorous, but keep your shoulders and arms tightly compact so that you do not over-swing and injure your joint. Begin slowly and make sure your arms are warm from other exercises before you attempt this one.

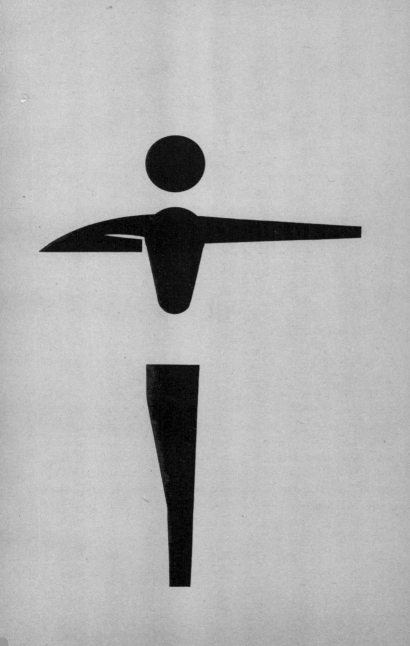